Flowers Blooming in Antartica

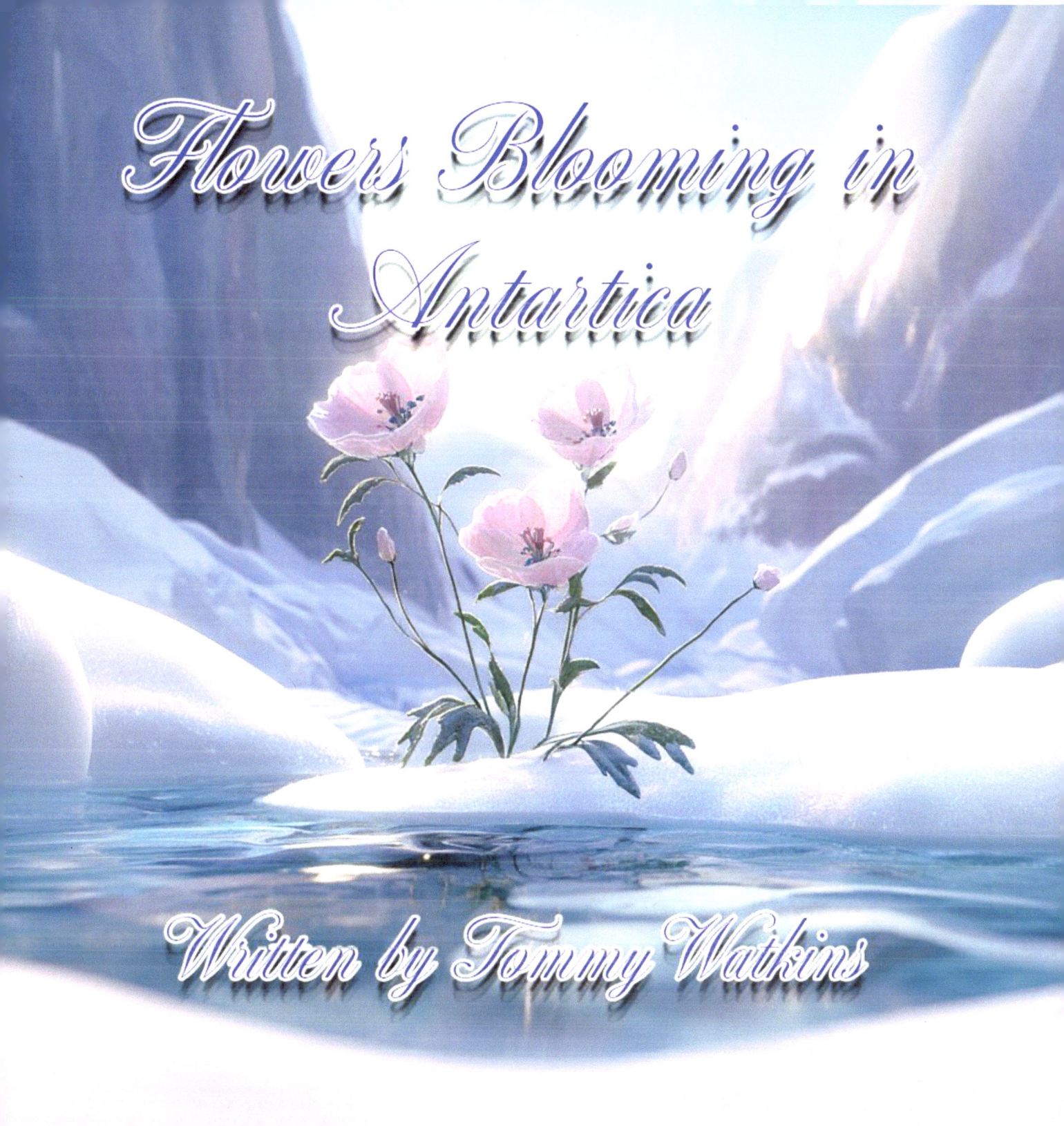

Written by Tommy Watkins

New Year's Day is tomorrow, and I'm ready for a fresh start.

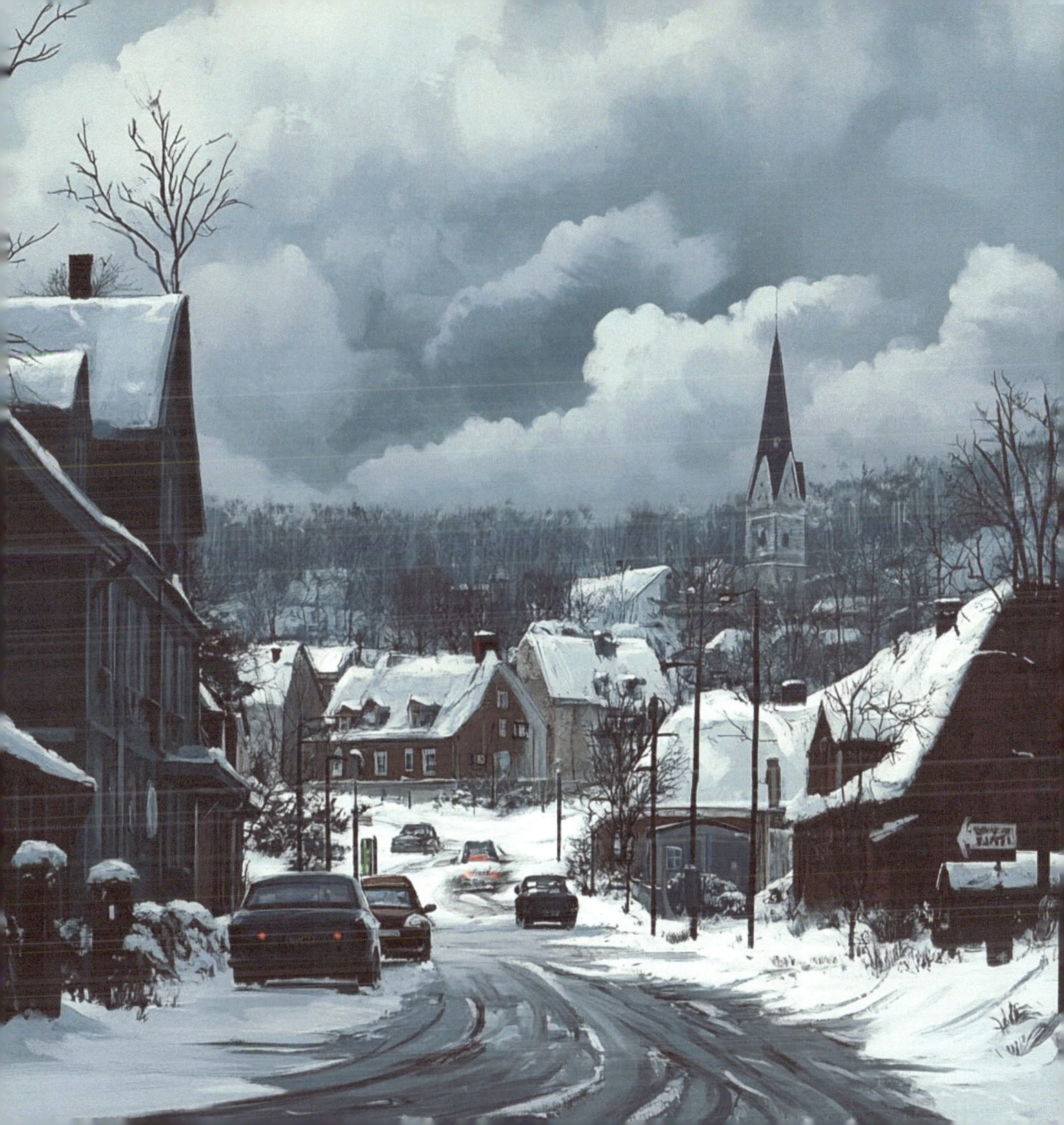

I don't have plans tonight, just a pizza, beer, and watching New Year's Fireworks on television.

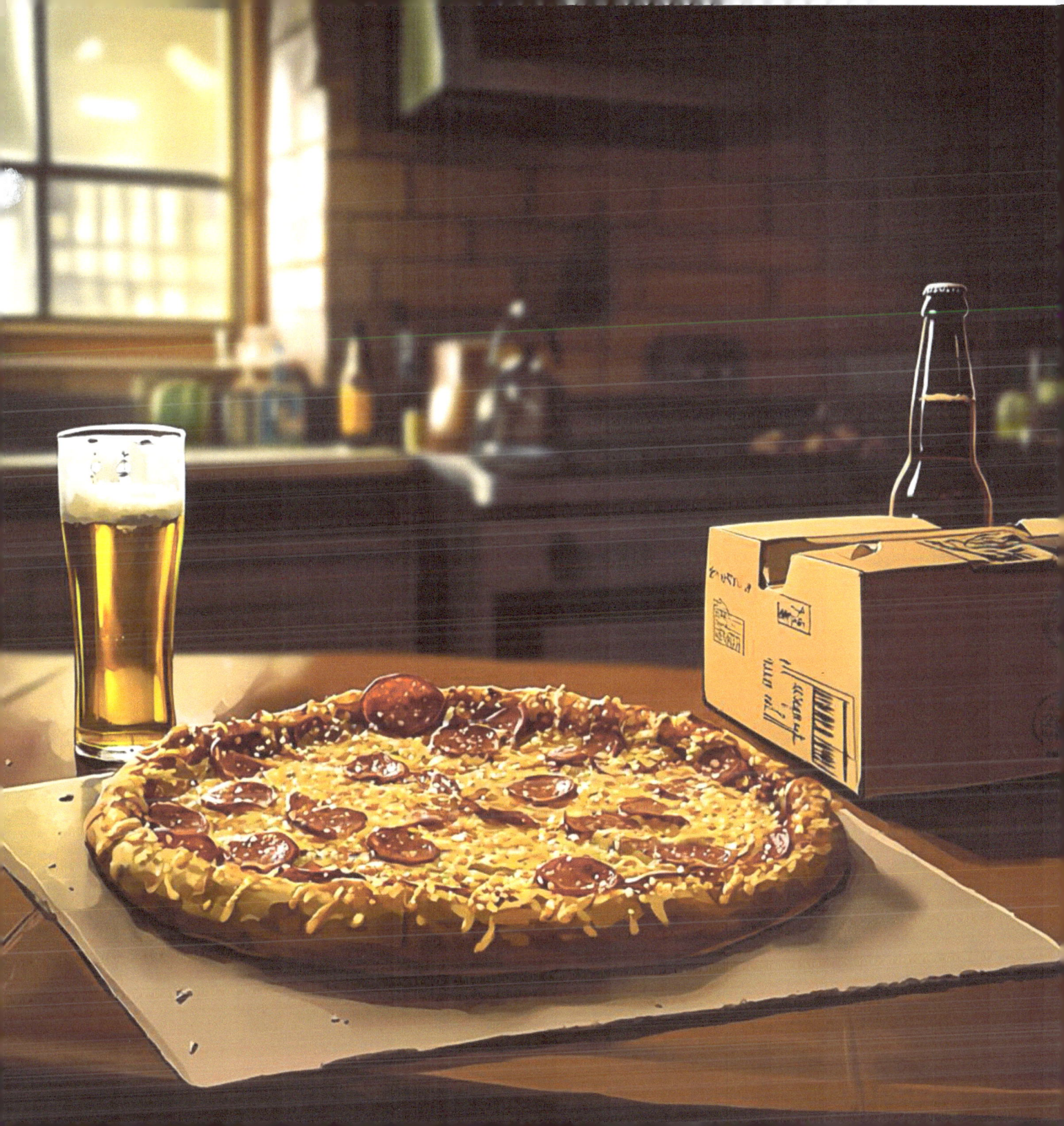

This year hasn't been my best. My attitude to others and my living habits, things could be better.

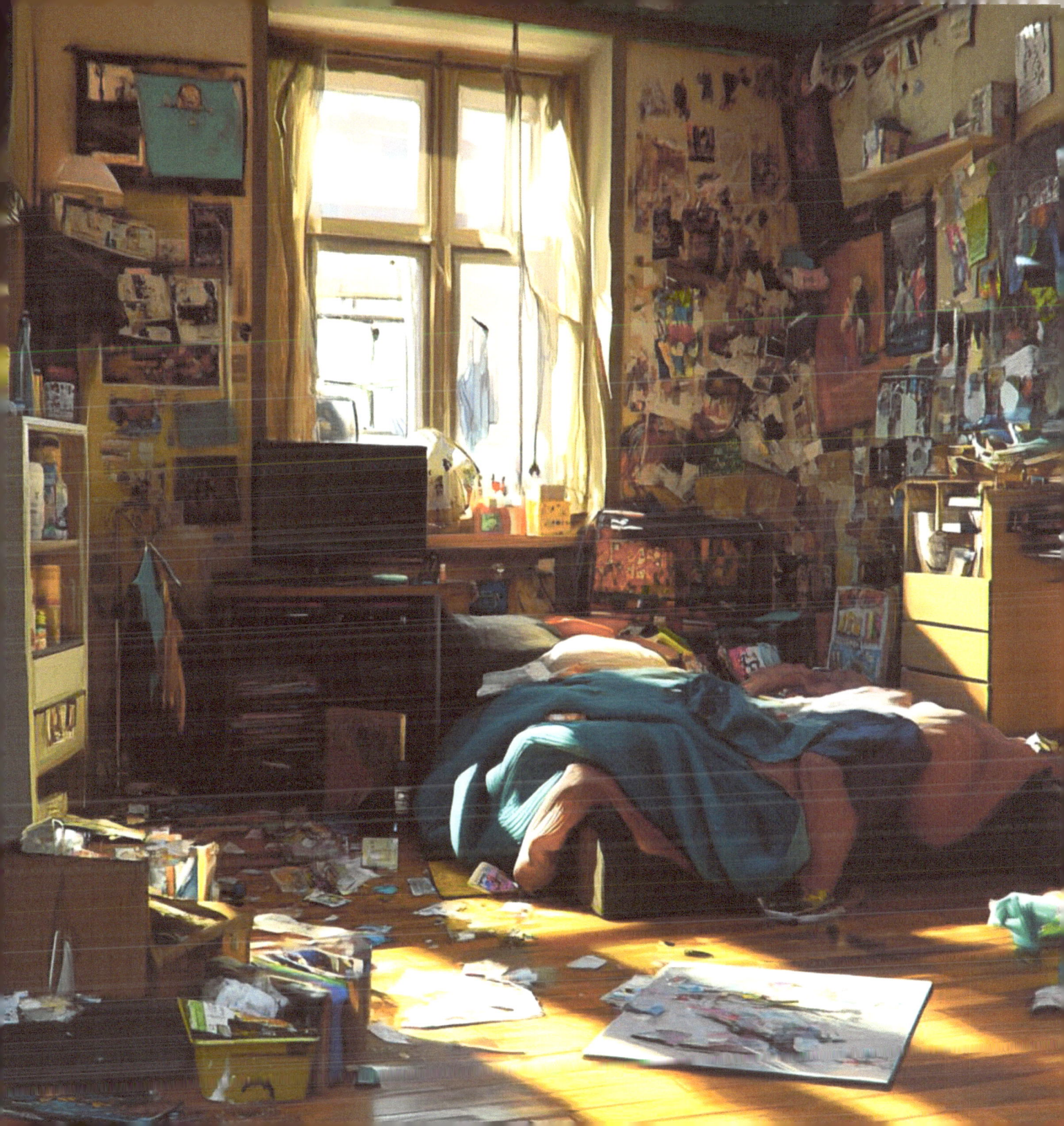

While I don't have a significant other to kiss at midnight. I can sulk in my beers and half-eaten pizza.

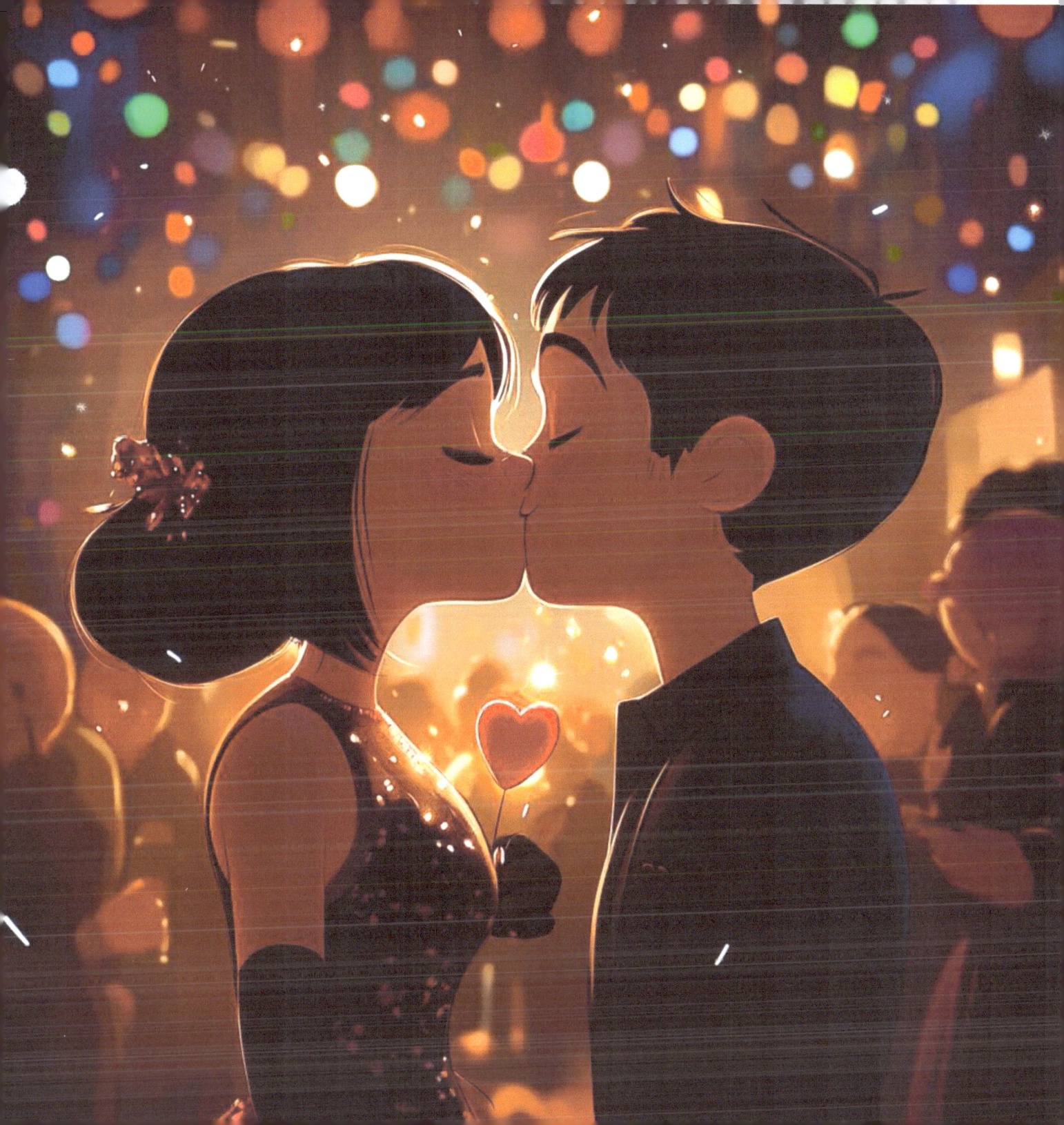

The clock hits 11:30 pm. I watch all the parties going on television. I'm through half my case of beer.

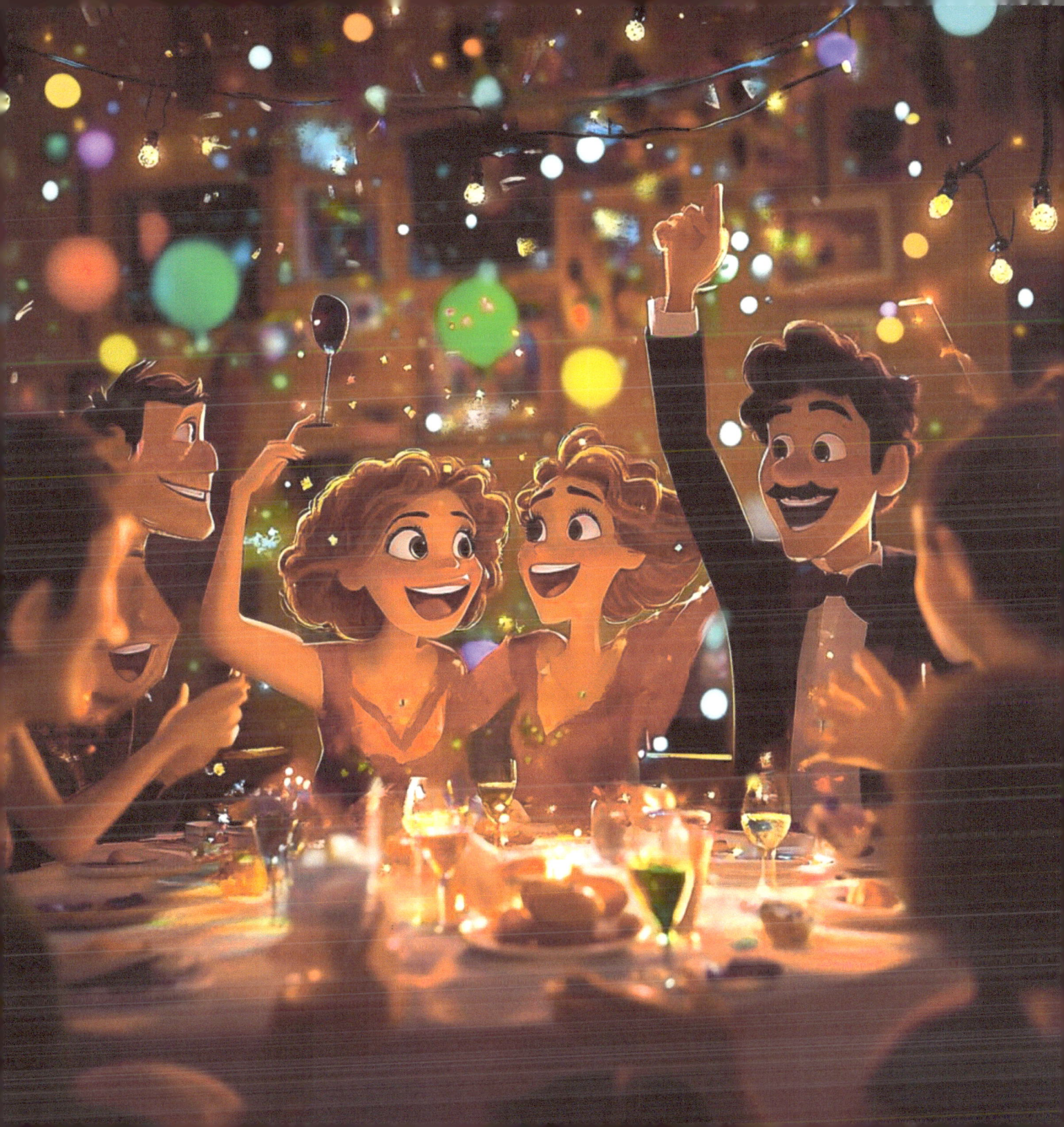

As I'm ready to go to sleep, the countdown brings. 5, 4, 3, 2, 1, Happy New Year!

Fireworks are going off outside my window.

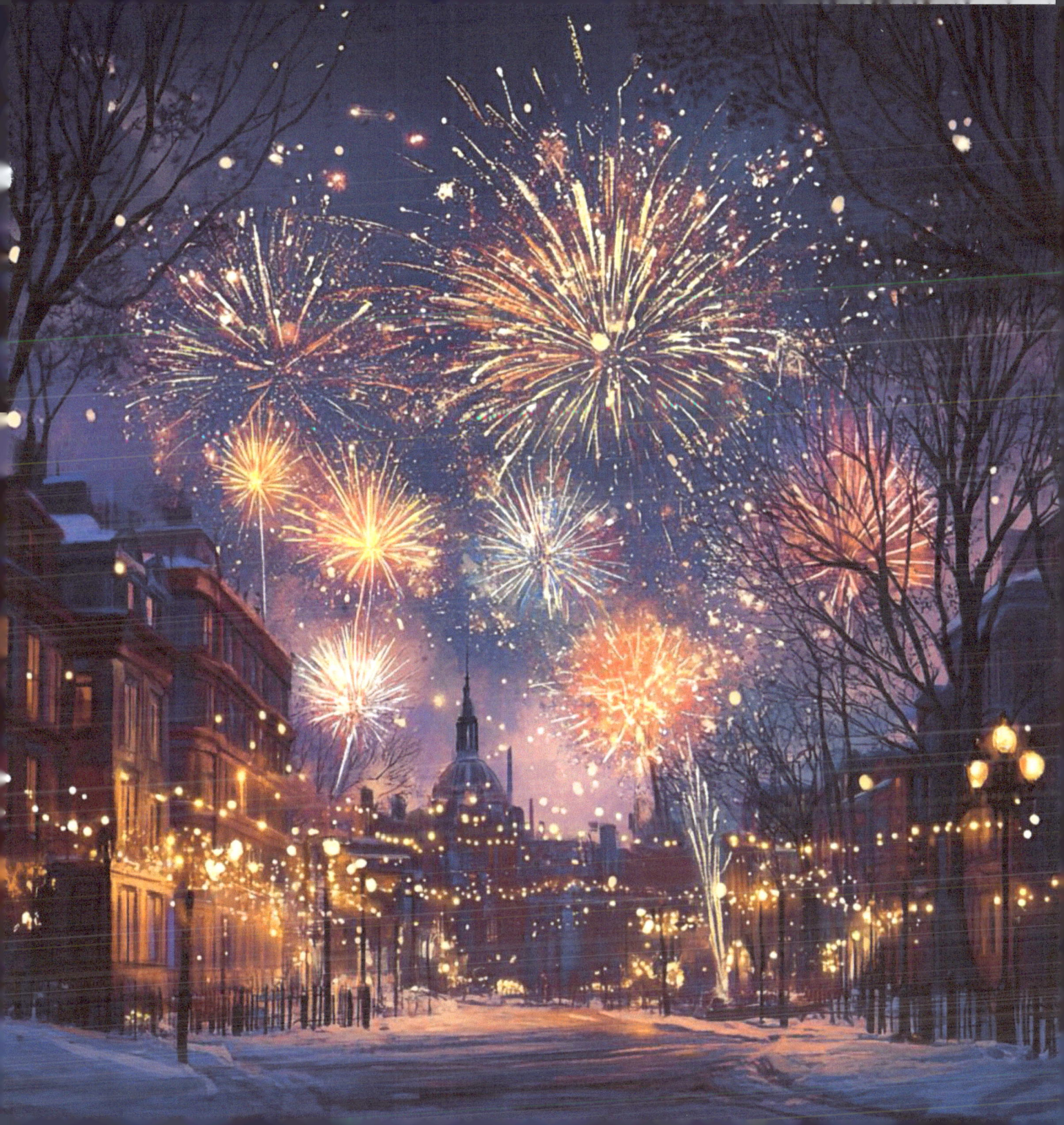

I think I can change and make my life better! I can be a better person, be productive, and have a significant other in my life.

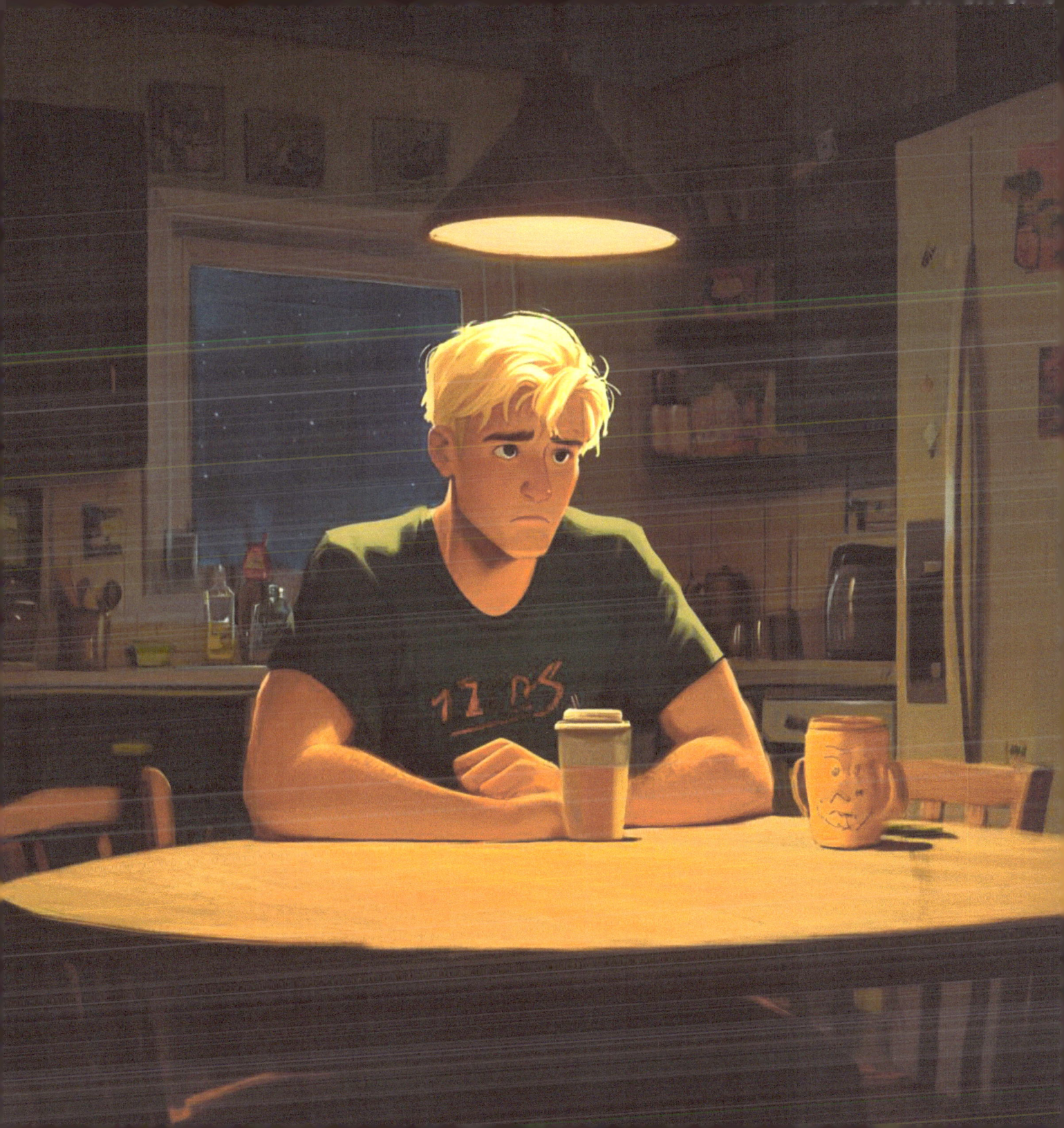

Or maybe it's just all the liquid courage talking, and I'll go back to drinking all the time.

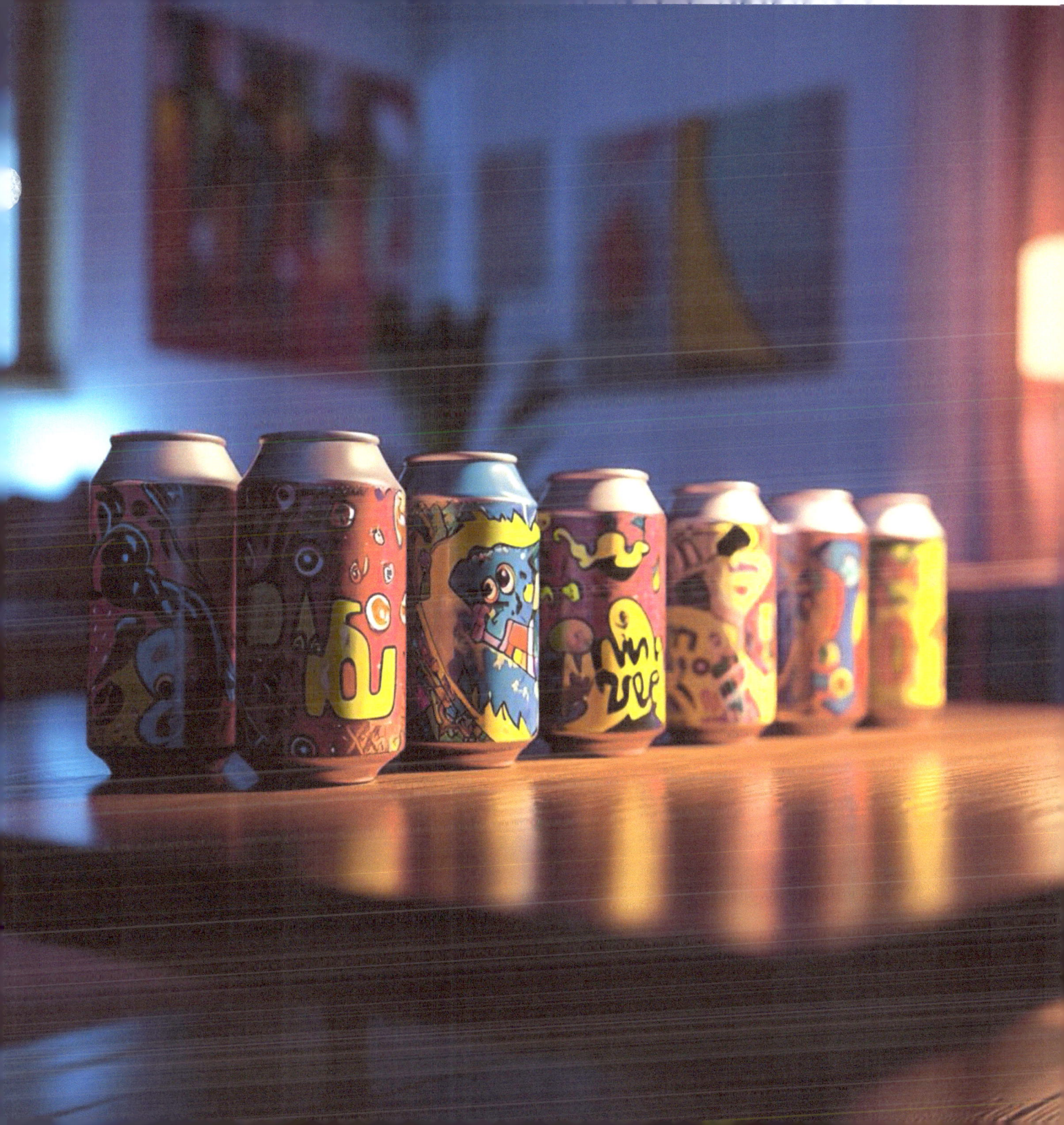

I can be like those flowers that bloom through the ice. Those flowers blooming in Antarctica. If they can bloom through ice, why can't I?

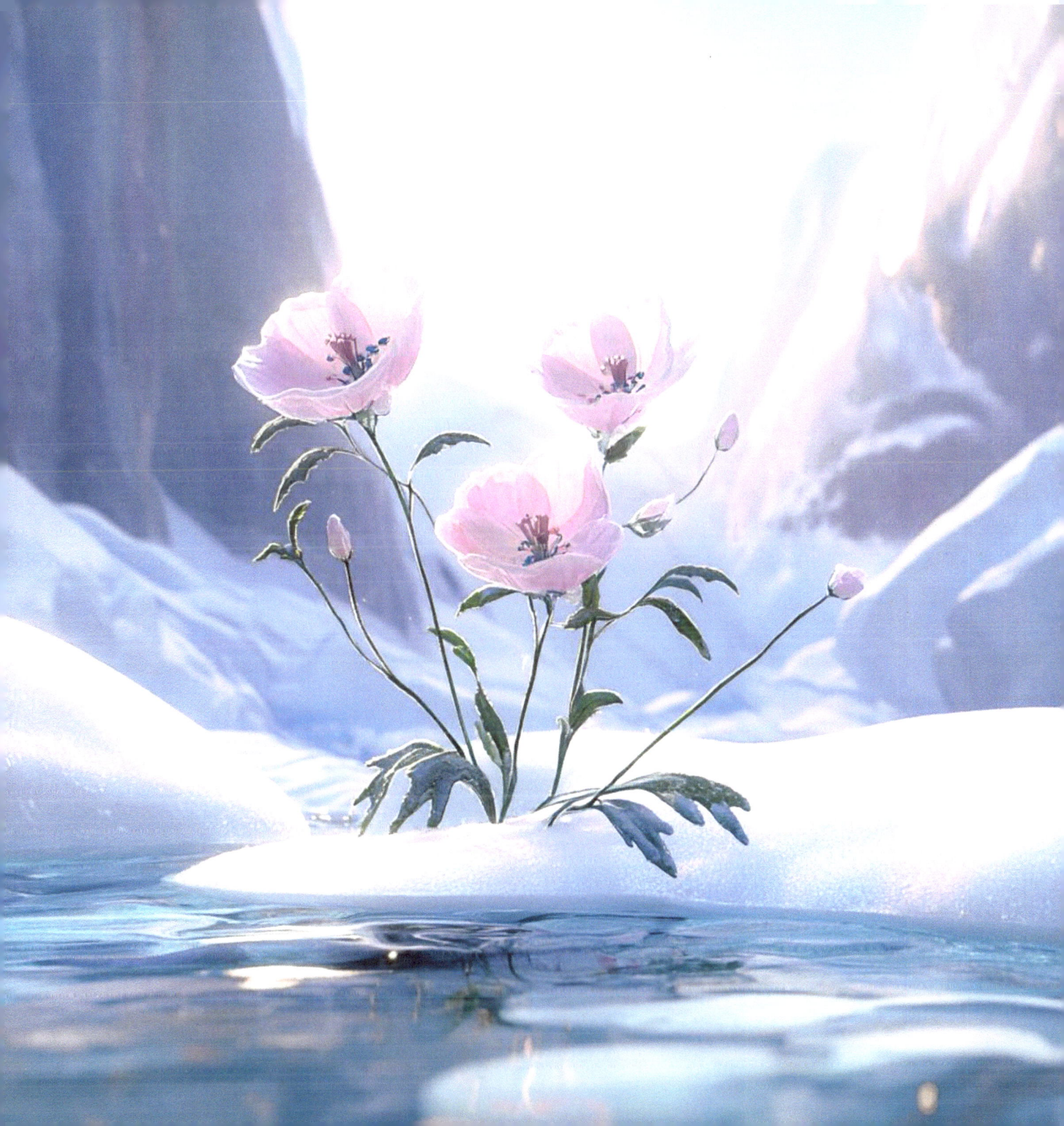

The End

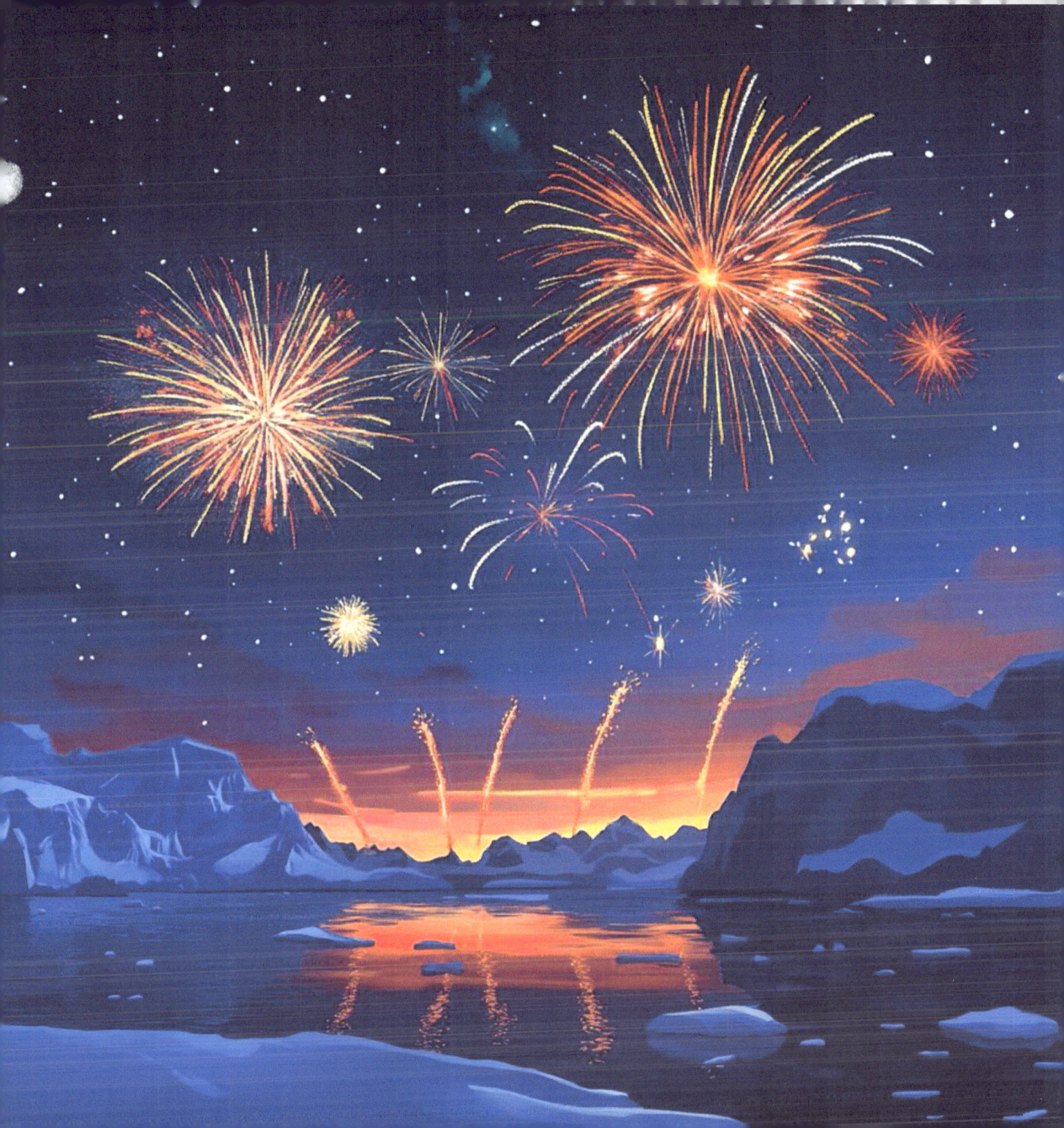